Clear
Skin

Heal Your Skin and End the
Breakouts Once and for All

CLEAR SKIN

HEAL YOUR SKIN

AND END THE BREAKOUTS

ONCE AND FOR ALL

Dan Kern

Introduction by Jerome Aronberg, M.D.

A Perigee Book

A Perigee Book
Published by The Berkley Publishing Group
A division of Penguin Group (USA) Inc.
375 Hudson Street
New York, New York 10014

First Perigee paperback edition: March 2004

ISBN: 0-399-52948-9

This book has been cataloged by the Library of Congress

Printed in the United States of America

10   9   8   7   6   5   4   3   2   1

For Deepak Chopra,
whose words inspired me to help others

CONTENTS

Acknowledgments   ix

Introduction by Jerome Aronberg, M.D.   xi

1. MY SKIN, MY STORY   1

2. GETTING UNDER YOUR SKIN:
   THE EMOTIONS SURROUNDING ACNE   11

3. THE BIOLOGY BEHIND THE DISEASE   21

4. GETTING CLEAR AND STAYING CLEAR:
   THE CLEAR SKIN REGIMEN   37

5. FREQUENTLY ASKED QUESTIONS   65

6. THE CLEAR PATH AHEAD   81

   SKIN CARE JOURNAL   104

ACKNOWLEDGMENTS

Sharing my Clear Skin regimen is my way of reaching out to people. I would like to acknowledge those individuals who allowed me to reach out to even more people by making this book a reality.

Thank you to Rachel Cagney for her invaluable contributions to the manuscript. Her way with words helped me produce the very book I had envisioned. My gratitude goes out to Karen Watts and her colleagues at Lark Productions, who believed in me and this project from the get-go. Thank you also to Lauren Kanter, whose creativity, enthusiasm, and editorial instincts helped guide this book from its earliest stages.

INTRODUCTION

Like many acne sufferers, Daniel Kern spent a long time searching for a treatment that would work for him. As a dermatologist, I know how desperate acne patients can be to clear up their skin. I have worked with many patients to find the treatment (or combination of treatments) that would improve their skin. It's not an easy process and it's rarely quick, thanks to the many variables each patient brings to the table.

The fact is, acne is a disease. It can range in scope and severity. *Acne mechanica,* acne that is induced by mechanical friction—such as forehead and chin acne caused by helmets and chin straps—may plague, for example, football or hockey players. *Acne tropicalis,* which is usually seen on the back, may affect people who live in very hot, humid locales. *Acne cosmetica* is induced by oils that are found in certain cosmetic products. These are some of the specific manifestations of acne that fall under the umbrella of *acne vulgaris*, or common acne, the mild to moderate garden-variety acne that plagues 70 million people at any given time.

Common acne is evidenced by blackheads and whiteheads (comedones), and/or red bumps and red-rimmed whiteheads (papules and pustules), present to varying degrees on different regions of the face. There are grades of common acne, which are determined by the number of lesions there are on a given side of the face, ranging from under ten (grade I) to more than thirty or fifty (grade IV), depending on whether they're comedones or papular lesions. It's important to understand that common acne is distinct from severe cystic acne, or *acne conglobata,* which is essentially beyond grading because it is so intense, pervasive, and active.

What Daniel Kern has discovered, from his own careful research and experience, is that benzoyl peroxide can be very effective in controlling lower-grade common acne. He experimented widely with the various concentrations of benzoyl peroxide (from 2.5 percent to 10 percent strengths) as well as the process of cleansing the skin and applying the benzoyl peroxide, and discovered an extremely effective regimen for people with lower-grade common acne like his. He figured out what dermatologists have known since the 1930s—benzoyl peroxide can act as a drying agent and a bacteriostatic agent, by releasing oxygen that essentially disables the bacterium that causes acne. What he figured out that dermatologists may *not* have known is that the powerful combination of a careful cleansing and treatment regimen and the use of generous quantities of 2.5 percent benzoyl peroxide is an over-the-counter alternative that can really work!

His Clear Skin regimen is not for folks with severe acne. It's for people with light to moderate acne who are prepared to carefully adhere to his step-by-step cleansing and treatment regimen. By working out this regimen and clearing up his own skin, he's done the hard work for you—the trial and error and experimenting on process and product that most people wouldn't be willing or able to do. His regimen is safe and simple, his reasoning is sound, and, as a dermatologist, I support his dream of helping others gain control of their acne through this book. The cost of trying the regimen is minimal; the value of its success if it works for you is priceless.

—Jerome Aronberg, M.D.

Clear Skin

Heal Your Skin and End the Breakouts Once and for All

1

MY SKIN, MY STORY

My own battle with acne started when I was eleven years old. I know from experience how devastating the effects of persistent acne can be—whether you've had it for two months or twenty years. Having acne doesn't just affect your skin, it affects your life—how you feel about yourself, how you interact with others, and all the time you spend obsessing about your skin. I know it often seems like you're the only one who feels this way, but the truth is that there are millions of people out there who share these same emotions. I am one of them. Let me tell you my story.

I remember my first zit—I was in the sixth grade.

It popped up right between my eyebrows. That one pimple was the beginning of my battle with acne. In response to my constant breakouts, I started scrubbing my skin with a washcloth three times a day and scrubbing further with Stridex pads to try to get rid of the pimples. After a year or so with little success after all that scrubbing, I discovered benzoyl peroxide and started using the 10 percent Oxy 10 brand of product. I'd use a bit and I wouldn't get as many new pimples, but my breakouts never stopped. All the while I continued to harshly scrub my face with a washcloth. What I didn't realize was that all that scrubbing was just making the situation worse.

When I reached high school I started seeing a dermatologist and began my cycle of different prescription medications. I started out by taking antibiotics faithfully for months with no results whatsoever. I moved on to Retin-A and found out that it made my acne worse—a whole lot worse—and unfortunately my acne never got better. Going to see a dermatologist wasn't a complete waste of time, however, because I learned two very important things about treating acne. The first was to wash my face only twice a day and the second was to be very gentle with my skin. These simple but important lessons are key elements of what would become my ultimate success with the Clear Skin regimen.

My skin continued to get worse as I entered college, often riddled with large lesions that lasted for weeks, and acne consistently broke out on my upper back. Desperate, I started doing some research on acne. I read a book that suggested treating acne with a lot of 10 percent benzoyl peroxide instead of the small amounts I had used in the past. The theory was that the benzoyl peroxide would dry out the skin, and then the skin and the pimples would peel off. I started smearing on a thick layer of the 10 percent benzoyl peroxide, and my face peeled, all right. My skin was uncontrollably dry and very red but the acne seemed a bit better, so I continued the fight. Even with all of this medication, though, my acne just wouldn't clear up, and now my skin was dry and itchy.

I continued to be desperate for a solution. I hit the books once more and I discovered a drug called Accutane. It seemed like a miracle—it promised to completely clear up acne and keep skin clear forever. It sounded like a plan to me, so I made an appointment with my dermatologist. But before she would prescribe Accutane, she wanted me to try another solution. At her suggestion, I started a cycle of a clindamycin medicine and sulfur. The sulfur smelled bad and was colored, so I looked like I was trying to use makeup to cover up the pimples. This treatment didn't work and my acne got increasingly worse.

One look at my skin after that clindamycin and sulfur fiasco and the dermatologist agreed to put me on Accutane. I waited eagerly for the results of the preliminary blood tests that would qualify me as a safe candidate for Accutane and finally got the okay to start the prescription. I took Accutane for the normal cycle (fifteen to twenty weeks) and amazingly, thrillingly, it worked. Within two or three weeks of starting with Accutane, I cleared up completely and had a great semester with acne-free skin. It was a dream come true. I was more outgoing and no longer felt I had to hide my face. Most of all, I was happy.

While on Accutane, I experienced severely dry skin and lips and had to use loads of moisturizer to keep it under control. It also caused all the joints in my body to ache, but I continued the treatment because finally having clear skin seemed worth the price

I was paying with the side effects. While I was on a semester abroad in London, my cycle of Accutane came to an end. Almost immediately, my skin began to break out again, first with a few minor spots, then returning to real acne within a few months. I was crushed. My acne wasn't as bad as it was before taking Accutane, but I was still plagued with breakouts. The dermatologist determined that my acne this time around wasn't bad enough for another cycle of Accutane, so I was stuck with acne again. Having finally known what life was like with clear skin, I dreaded the thought of going back to life with chronic acne.

I started looking for another solution in earnest, so I went back to what had worked somewhat in the past—benzoyl peroxide. I started up again with the 10 percent benzoyl peroxide, but this time I used less to keep my skin from becoming overly dry and red. I also continued to use moisturizer and that seemed to help with the dryness. Then I found a 5 percent benzoyl peroxide at the drugstore that claimed to work as well as the 10 percent solution, without overly drying the skin. I bought it. This lower dosage seemed to work well, but I still had a few pimples to deal with every day. I used this formula for a few years and resigned myself to the fact that I'd have some acne forever. I was still washing gently, trying not to irritate my skin and this helped to keep the acne somewhat under control. And I continued to moisturize every day to prevent dryness.

One day, I thought about my earlier experience with using loads of 10 percent benzoyl peroxide. It dawned on me that I might be able to use lots of the 5 percent solution the same way, but this time combined with moisturizer to keep my skin from becoming so dry and red. I faithfully applied three times the amount of benzoyl peroxide than I had been using and, lo and behold, my skin started to clear up. Bolstered by this success, I continued and my skin kept getting clearer. After a few days it was completely clear, and it stayed that way. I still found the 5 percent benzoyl peroxide solution overly drying, so I switched to a 2.5 percent solution and before too long, my skin was clear and balanced. I had finally found the key. I fiddled with the formula of washing, applying benzoyl peroxide, and moisturizing until I found a combination of products and procedures that cleared up my face—for good. I still get an isolated zit from time to time, but it is usually small and of little consequence. In other words, it's perfectly normal and no one would ever suspect that I had ever had an acne problem.

After all the years I spent trying to clear up my skin, I discovered two things that are the basis of the Clear Skin regimen—benzoyl peroxide does a great job of killing acne bacteria, and irritating your skin makes your acne worse.

2

GETTING UNDER YOUR SKIN: THE EMOTIONS SURROUNDING ACNE

Even though I found a way to clear up my own skin, I've never forgotten what it was like to live with chronic acne. Desperately trying to get rid of it, I tried everything under the sun. I was frustrated by the lack of results and angry because I'd wasted time and money on yet another dead end. I'm here to tell you that the anxiety you feel about your acne is indeed very real. Here are some of the common emotions that people experience when they live with acne. I have a feeling that you'll relate to at least some of them, if not all of them.

Anger

When you're plagued by acne, you're angry at everything. You're mad at the advertisers whose empty
promises have left your wallet thinner and your hopes
dashed. You fume when you think about people who
have commented on or even appeared to notice your
complexion. You're angry at the celebrities who
make looking good so easy. You want to scream when
you think about all those dollars and hours you've
wasted visiting doctors and trying costly yet ineffec-
tive products. But the worst part is, you're angry at
yourself. Why, of all people, do *you* have this devastating problem? Why can't you just clear it up? Why
are you always on the losing side of this battle against
acne?

Depression

Having acne *can* be a factor leading to feelings of depression. All you can think about is your acne, and

when it doesn't go away, you find yourself sliding into feelings of hopelessness and despair. Some people actually get so depressed about their acne they think about suicide. While that may seem extreme, the reality is that the depression you feel from having acne is real and can affect every aspect of your life.

Depression is more than just feeling a little down. It's a serious condition where you can't get rid of your feelings of sadness and hopelessness. Some symptoms of depression can include changes in your eating and/or sleeping habits, lasting feelings of sadness, trouble concentrating, lethargy, loss of interest in activities you previously found enjoyable, and thoughts of suicide or death. Depression shouldn't be ignored and a trip to your doctor or other health professional may be in order to help treat your depression.

Desperation

This is the "I'll try anything" response to having acne. You've tried a lot of things but nothing worked. You've gone on to the next thing, then the next, and on and on. You spend lots of money, try many different products, and listen to a lot of bad advice along the way. Clear skin eludes you, but you keep experimenting in the hopes you'll find that magic solution.

Believe me, I've been there. Many people spend years in this horrendous cycle of trying this and that, just to be repeatedly frustrated when their acne doesn't clear up. So much time and energy is spent obsessing about your skin and how to fix it—time you won't be able to get back.

Frustration

You've done it all—acne treatments, avoiding certain foods, scrubbing your face hard every day—but you still can't control your acne. You figure that there is something wrong with you because you can't even clear up your own skin. Your parents or friends try to help with suggestions, but you've truly given it all you've got and you still can't win the battle with your acne. You may even feel that people with clear skin are getting ahead of you in school or work because you're perceived as lacking determination or commitment because you can't control your acne. People without acne just don't understand that you really work hard to get rid of it—it's just that nothing works.

Negative Self-Image

You cringe when you look in the mirror—if you can even look at all. You feel ugly. Sometimes you think there's no reason to bother with your appearance, since it's not going to help disguise your acne. Your inability to fix this problem makes you feel down about yourself. You try to disappear so no one will notice you or your acne.

Resignation

There may come a point where you figure that you've got acne, and that's that. Nothing is going to change the fact that you've got acne-infested skin because you've tried every possible solution and none of it has worked. You think that this is the best that it's going to get—the best *you're* going to get. You feel like you're going to look like this forever, so you might as well get used to it. You know it's a cop-out, but it's easier than continuing to fight a losing battle.

Self-Consciousness

Having an acne problem can make you think that your pimples are all that everyone else can see. Because that's all *you* can see. When people make remarks about your skin (nasty or sympathetic) you see it as confirmation that your acne stands out more than anything else about you.

All of this can make you hide—physically and emotionally. You try to cover your face with a hairstyle or avoid looking people in the eye. You stay away from social situations so you don't have to show your face. You're embarrassed to be out in public so you withdraw from life because it's easier to do that than to confront the world with your bad skin.

For everyone who has ever had any of these feelings about themselves and their acne, I want to share the Clear Skin regimen with you. After my success in clearing up my own skin, I decided that I wanted to help other people do the same. I was inspired by the

Who Should Use the Clear Skin Method ▪

The Clear Skin regimen works for people with mild to moderate acne. In general, mild and moderate acne are defined by the different types of acne a person has on their skin. Mild acne consists of only whiteheads and blackheads. Moderate acne is characterized by the existence of papules and pustules, which are small, reddish bumps, as well as whiteheads and blackheads. People with severe acne—those with nodules and cysts—should see a dermatologist for acne treatments. A more complete discussion of the degrees of acne can be found in chapter 3.

philosophy of Deepak Chopra, who said that every individual has a unique way of helping others. Sharing my success is *my* way of helping people in their search for clear skin and self-confidence. I am confident that the Clear Skin regimen will work when followed carefully and precisely. You don't have to live with acne.

3

THE BIOLOGY BEHIND
THE DISEASE

The first thing you have to understand is that acne is a disease. It isn't the result of dirty skin or something you ate. There are, however, certain factors that can aggravate acne, and it is important for you to be aware of these things, because while acne can't be cured, it can be managed. These are all facts about acne that you need to know to start the process of clearing up your skin. How acne starts is also valuable information in your quest for clear skin, so let's first look at how your skin works—from the way it's supposed to operate to how acne actually develops.

What Is Acne?

Acne is the result of a blocked pore. To understand exactly how acne starts, you first need to become familiar with how your skin works. Tiny hair follicles—commonly called pores—are the source of all the activity. Located at the base of the follicle are sebaceous glands. These glands produce sebum, or oil, that travels up the follicle. This sebum is released at the surface of the skin. Normally, this is a smooth process, but when something inhibits the oil from reaching the surface—voila, you've got the beginning of acne.

The problem starts when the walls of the pore stick together. The sebaceous glands keep producing the oil, but it's got no outlet to the surface. As the oil builds up at the base of the follicle, bacteria (*Propionibacterium acnes*) starts to grow in that blocked pore. *This* is the start of acne.

Types of Acne

The Clear Skin regimen is effective for people with *light to moderate acne,* which consists of whiteheads, blackheads, papules, pustules, or a combination of all of them. *Severe acne* is categorized by the appearance of nodules and cysts in combination with papules and pustules.

Whiteheads vs. Blackheads

Both whiteheads and blackheads—called comedones—are forms of acne. The difference between the two is where the actual blockage ends up—just under the skin's surface (whiteheads) or actually opening to the surface (blackheads).

When the sebum blockage remains beneath the skin, the bacteria continue to multiply. When the walls of the follicle finally open up, all of the trapped sebum and bacteria get pushed up toward the surface of the skin, producing a whitehead.

Blackheads occur when this same discharge of sebum, bacteria, and white blood cells is only partially blocked. The blockage reaches the skin's surface and looks black against the skin—thus the term blackhead.

Papules

Light to moderate acne is defined by the presence of papules and pustules, or inflammatory acne. Papules are small, solid pink/red bumps on the skin. These raised bumps remain beneath the surface and are apt to scar.

Pustules

Pustules are your garden-variety inflamed whitehead—an elevated, pus-filled comedone with a white or yellow head and red edges.

Nodules and Cysts

Nodules and Cysts are the characteristics that define a case of "severe" acne. Nodules are large, solid lesions deep within the skin. These lesions are often painful and may be visible as large red bumps on the skin. Nodules can last for months and can lead to scarring. Cysts are pus-filled lesions located deep within the skin. Cysts are most often very painful and can cause scarring. People with severe acne should see a dermatologist for treatment to reduce scarring.

Are They Even Zits?

Rosacea, rashes, and boils can often be confused with acne. All can appear similar to acne, but will not respond to acne treatments. Rosacea is a facial disease that makes the center of the face (cheeks, nose, chin, and sometimes the forehead) look like it has a red rash. Acne may occur in the presence of rosacea, complicating the diagnosis and requiring separate treatments for each condition. Rashes and boils may look like acne—red bumps or pus-filled lesions—but also will not respond to acne treatments. A doctor can determine by examination exactly what the condition is and recommend an appropriate treatment for either the rash or the boil.

Who Gets Acne?

Acne is usually considered an adolescent problem. Studies show that up to 90 percent of adolescents will at some point develop acne, but for many people, the problem can persist into adulthood. Even babies and the elderly can get acne. While there are no sure insights as to who will get acne, one of the major indicators is heredity. If your parents had acne problems, you're more likely to have the same condition. The gene that causes acne is a dominant gene—meaning that it's more likely than not that you'll inherit the gene from either or both of your parents.

Factors That Worsen Acne

Sometimes you can actually make your acne worse by some of the things that you do. Other times, your acne may get worse from either medicines you're taking or plain old hormones over which you have no control. Being aware of these situations can help you manage your acne, or at least help you understand why your breakouts seem worse.

Harsh Washcloths

Scrubbing with washcloths irritates the skin, which can worsen your acne. While it's tempting to try to scrub away the problem, a gentle approach to cleansing your skin is best. While you're in the process of trying to clear up your face, you want your skin to heal, and constant irritation doesn't promote healing. Keeping your skin clear requires a delicate touch.

Constant Picking

Letting your skin heal from breakouts is a necessary part of managing your acne. When you pick at healing pimples, you're inhibiting your skin's ability to restore itself. Scabs are a protective layer, shielding an open sore from the outside world. Skin heals from the inside out, so when you pull off that protective scab, your skin has to start the healing process all over again. Picking at those spots can also cause scarring, which is something you want to try to avoid.

Don't pick! ■

Not only does picking at your pimples prohibit healing, the picking itself is irritating to the skin. Constantly rubbing and scratching aggravates acne-prone skin.

Changing Hormone Levels

Unfortunately, this is usually something that you can't control. Adolescents often experience flare-ups due to hormonal changes, which may seem to happen constantly. Pregnant women, premenstrual women, and menopausal women may also experience bouts of acne due to their changing levels of hormones. While these hormonal changes can't be stopped, it does explain why your breakouts are worse at some times than others.

Friction

Helmets, backpacks, or tight collars rubbing against the skin can trigger flare-ups. Frequent use of the telephone can also worsen acne in areas where the receiver touches the skin, such as the chin or cheekbone areas. Leaning your face in your hands isn't any good for your acne either. When you prop your head up by placing your cheek or forehead against your hand, the friction caused from skin rubbing against skin can irritate your acne. You should strive to keep your face untouched.

Environmental Irritants

Pollution and humidity can aggravate your already irritated skin. Prolonged exposure to petroleum products and cooking oils can also make your acne worse.

Medication

Some medications—especially certain antidepressants, hormones, and lithium—have increased acne as a side effect. Discuss this side effect with your doctor so you can be prepared to treat your acne if it does occur because of your medication.

Cosmetics

Many cosmetics on the market are comedogenic, which means acne-causing. Certain facial makeup, sunscreens, self-tanners, and hair products can contribute to flare-ups.

Acne Myths

There is so much misinformation out there relating to acne—and you've probably heard it all. Some of this information has literally been passed down through generations, so it's commonly believed—whether it's been proven or not. Here are some common myths about what may cause acne and what may cure it.

Myth: Acne is related to diet.

Reality: Chocolate, potato chips, French fries, and other greasy (and good-tasting!) foods are all supposed to cause acne. They don't. There isn't any scientific information that proves there is a correlation between eating these foods and an increase in acne. Having said that, however, it's in your skin's best interest to eat a well-balanced diet to keep everything in tip-top shape. The good news is that if you eat a piece of chocolate birthday cake today, it will not become a zit tomorrow.

Myth: Lots of face washing will cure acne.

Reality: Washing your face more and harder *will not* clear up acne. Acne isn't caused by dirty skin, so washing it ten times a day isn't going to do you any good. Frequent washing and scrubbing with a washcloth actually irritates the skin, which can make your acne even worse.

Myth: Stress causes acne.

Reality: The debate about whether stress increases the occurrence of acne isn't over yet. Some people may experience an acne flare-up when stressed, but other people under the same type of stress won't suffer an increase in acne at all. It could be that being nervous or stressed causes you to touch or pick at your face more, so your acne worsens from that irritation; that would be indirectly related to stress. If you're one of those people who seems to have stress-related acne, take a deep breath, because constantly worrying about it will only make it worse.

Myth: Sex and masturbation cause acne.

Reality: There is no scientific research that shows that either sex or masturbation has *anything* to do with acne. Actually, this myth dates back to the sixteenth century (obviously acne is an age-old problem!), when it was believed that excess semen excretion aggravated acne. It was said, too, that acne cleared up after marriage. This myth was likely created to discourage people from masturbating or having premarital sex.

Myth: The sun is good for acne.

Reality: Exposure to the sun can create temporary skin redness, making the red acne spots blend into the sun-exposed skin tone. It has also been shown that sun exposure can help heal existing pimples. Both of these effects sound great, until you look at the big picture of sun exposure. A suntan is actually the skin's natural reaction to sun *damage*. Every time you tan, the sun is actually aggravating your skin, and we know that irritated skin can cause acne flare-ups. Acne can increase in the weeks following sun exposure as a reaction to this irritation. The truth is that the short-term benefits of sun exposure are outweighed by the future breakouts and skin damage that are likely to follow.

So now you're armed with real information about acne. The biology behind acne is pretty simple—your pores close up, bacteria grows, and acne is formed. Lots of people are likely to get acne. Your skin can react to all kinds of stimuli—but not some of the ones that you think. Many of the old acne myths are still around today, plaguing you with guilt every time you look in the mirror and see your acne, or giving you false hope for a cure. The bottom line is that understanding how acne develops, taking care not to irritate your skin, and knowing what does and doesn't cause acne form the foundation of your new acne line of defense.

4

GETTING CLEAR AND STAYING CLEAR: THE CLEAR SKIN REGIMEN

$$x + y + z = \text{Clear Skin}$$

As you're painfully aware, the mysterious values of x, y, and z are more difficult to solve than any calculus problem. I plugged in different values for x, y, and z from the time I spotted my first pimple in sixth grade until just after I graduated from college. Unfortunately, I could never seem to balance the equation.

As I explained in chapter 1, of all the treatments I tried—and there were plenty—I had the most success with benzoyl peroxide, the key ingredient in many over-the-counter acne products on the market.

When I graduated from college, benzoyl peroxide was the most effective treatment I had tried so far. Yet while my skin responded well to it and did improve with repeated use, I couldn't prevent the acne from reoccurring. Finding myself so close to a solution but falling short was just painful.

As I looked at myself in the mirror one fine day, I exclaimed, "That's it! I'm loading this benzoyl peroxide on! What do I have to lose except a few dollars?" I applied the benzoyl peroxide generously, about three times the amount I usually applied. "Ecstatic" isn't strong enough to describe how I felt when after three or four days, my skin was remarkably clear.

Many tests and trials later, I had modified the cleansing and medicating regimen, and today, seven years later, I still don't need to worry about acne when I look in the mirror.

The values of $x,$ $y,$ and z? They don't elude me anymore. I've balanced the equation:

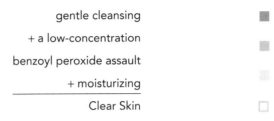

gentle cleansing
+ a low-concentration
benzoyl peroxide assault
+ moisturizing
_____
Clear Skin

Clearly Benzoyl

So what makes benzoyl peroxide so special? The secret is in the way it attacks acne. Benzoyl peroxide is *the best* OTC or prescription medication for killing the bacterium (*P. acnes*) that is fundamental to the growth of a pimple. The benzoyl peroxide is applied to the surface of the skin, but it gets down into the pore— where it creates oxygen. Now, here's the clincher—the bacterium won't survive in the presence of oxygen, so when the oxygen created by the benzoyl peroxide gets into the pore, the *P. acnes* is killed right where it lives. Benzoyl peroxide also has some mild drying and peeling effects, which may further help clear up your skin.

Benzoyl peroxide treatments come in strengths up to 10 percent. The percentage refers to the amount of active ingredient (benzoyl peroxide) in the product. Naturally, you'd think that if benzoyl peroxide works so well, you'd want the highest percentage you can get. Wrong. The higher the percentage of benzoyl peroxide, the more irritating it is to your skin. Your goal is to get the benefit of the benzoyl peroxide without the skin irritation, so I recommend the lowest percentage—2.5 percent—for use with the Clear Skin regimen. Studies show that the 2.5 percent works just as well as the higher percentages, but you won't suffer from the severe overdrying and redness that can occur when a more potent benzoyl peroxide product is used. You're going to be using *a lot* of benzoyl peroxide on the Clear Skin regimen, so the 2.5 percent solution is ideal.

Getting Ready to Get Clear

I don't promote specific brands; instead, I recommend a few products and encourage you to experiment with them and note the way your skin responds. No one knows your skin better than you do, so select the brand that you find works best for you.

PRODUCT CHECKLIST:

☐ *Cleanser.* Choose a cleanser that does not overdry. You want a mild formula made specifically for sensitive and dry skin. Make sure your cleanser does not contain any acne medications, such as salicylic acid, sulfur, resorcinol, or even benzoyl peroxide. You will be using *a lot* of benzoyl peroxide and your skin will deserve some TLC from a gentle cleanser!

☐ *Moisturizer.* Skin treated with the amount of benzoyl peroxide that I recommend demands moisture! It is vitally important that you begin moisturizing from day one, even if your skin doesn't appear to be thirsting for it. There are many quality moisturizers available that do not aggravate acne-prone skin, and applying them will help keep your skin in balance and prevent some of the initial drying effects of benzoyl peroxide. Look for an oil-free formula made especially for the face. Also, use a moisturizer that is SPF 15 or greater because you always want to be protecting your skin from the damaging effects of the sun.

□ *Low-concentration (2.5 percent) benzoyl peroxide cream or gel.*

Word to the Wise!

It may take your skin a couple of weeks to get used to benzoyl peroxide used in this quantity, especially if you've never used it before. With this fact in mind, you'll want to carefully follow the instructions for beginning the regimen and slowly increase the dosage as you continue with the treatment. While some redness and itchiness are normal at first, starting the regimen with such a large amount of benzoyl peroxide practically guarantees overly dry skin. If you start by using too much benzoyl peroxide, you may have to stop the regimen completely for a few days due to severe redness and dryness. *So start slowly!*

Also keep in mind that about 3 percent of people are allergic to benzoyl peroxide and may experience severe swelling and crusting. It's a good idea to test a spot on your face before you begin the regimen. If you experience swelling or crusting on your test area, stop using the benzoyl peroxide immediately and consult a doctor.

Recommended Brands

With the plethora of products available, a walk down the drug-store aisle can be incredibly daunting. But armed with this list of products that have worked for me, you can navigate the pharmacy with confidence.

Cleansers: Men should choose a bar (for its lather qualities while shaving); women may select a bar or a liquid cleanser.

- Purpose Gentle Cleansing Bar (6 oz.)
- Basic Sensitive Skin Bar (5.3 oz.)
- Purpose Gentle Cleansing Wash (6 oz.)
- Cetaphil Gentle Cleansing Bar, Unscented (4.5 oz.)
- Cetaphil Gentle Cleansing Bar, Antibacterial (4.5 oz.)
- Cetaphil Gentle Skin Cleanser Wash (4 oz., 8 oz., or 16 oz.)

Moisturizers: All the ones listed here are SPF 15 and come in a 4-ounce package. I recommend starting with one of the first three products listed below; alpha hydroxy formulas work great with benzoyl peroxide to prevent flakiness, but may sting if used when you first begin the regimen. After a few weeks, you can switch to an alpha hydroxy moisturizer.

- Neutrogena Oil-Free Moisture SPF 15
- Cetaphil Daily Facial Moisturizer
- Purpose Dual Treatment Moisture Lotion
- Eucerin Renewal Alpha Hydroxy Lotion

Benzoyl peroxide: Currently, there is only one 2.5 percent solution widely available on American drugstore shelves without a prescription.

- Neutrogena On-the-Spot Acne Treatment (0.75 oz.)

Visit my website (www.acne.org) regularly for news of larger, more economically sized packages of 2.5 percent benzoyl peroxide products. While none are currently available, I am working hard at lobbying companies to make a larger size.

I'm sure you're eager to begin, but there's one more thing to keep in mind as you go through the steps each day: *Follow the regimen as outlined!* When people have come to me upset that they have not achieved success, most of the time it is because they have not followed the regimen in some way. If you follow my method precisely, you should experience dramatic clearing.

To help you stick with the program and track your daily progress, I've included a Skin Care Journal at the end of this book.

The Clear Skin Regimen

Morning

1. Wash your face and any other problem areas (such as your back, chest, or neck) with the lather from a gentle cleansing bar or wash in the shower, using your bare hands—a washcloth will irritate. Your hands should barely touch your skin. Wash for only ten seconds or so to prevent irritation to the skin. Rinse with warm water. Washing this gently may seem very strange compared to how you may have scrubbed in the past, but remember, dirt does not cause acne and scrubbing the skin's surface does harm, not good.

2. Very gently pat (don't rub) dry with a towel. It's fine if your face is still a little damp.

3. Wait fifteen minutes for your skin to air-dry completely.

4. Wash and dry your hands.

5. This step changes during the first several weeks and refers to amounts of benzoyl peroxide to be used on the face only. Proportionate amounts should be used on other problem areas, such as the back, chest, or neck.

■ *Week one*—Squeeze out a small amount of benzoyl peroxide cream, as shown in figure 1. Use this amount of benzoyl peroxide at every application for a full week.

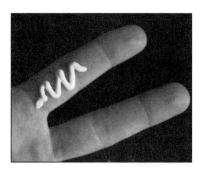

■ *Week two*—Squeeze out a larger amount of benzoyl peroxide cream, as shown in figure 2. Use this amount of benzoyl peroxide at every application for a full week.

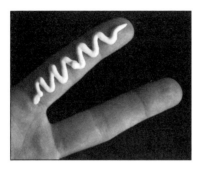

■ *Week three*—Squeeze out an even larger amount of benzoyl peroxide cream, as shown in figure 3. Use this amount of benzoyl peroxide at every application for a full week.

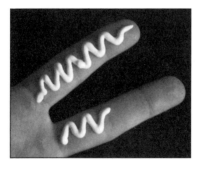

■ *Week four and beyond*—Squeeze out a *generous* portion of benzoyl peroxide cream onto your index finger. Squeeze out a *generous* portion. Squeeze out a *generous* portion. I say this three times because it is the most important step you will take!

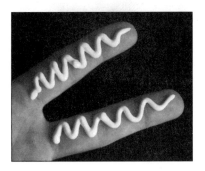

6. Using your other index finger, dab the cream in several spots around your problem areas. Work on one area at a time. Start with your right cheek, move on to your chin, then your left cheek, your forehead, and finally your nose. Doing one area at a time allows the benzoyl peroxide to be absorbed by the skin, not just drying on the surface. Then *gently* (and patiently) spread the cream into your skin with your fingertips. Be so gentle that you can hardly see the skin move beneath your fingers when applying. The benzoyl peroxide needs to be absorbed to prevent sticky white residue on the skin, but don't rub—you will only cause irrita-

tion. Carefully coat your entire problem area with the solution, not just the pimples themselves. *Do not apply benzoyl peroxide to the sensitive skin around the eyes.* You may experience severe redness if benzoyl peroxide comes in contact with the thin skin in the eye area.

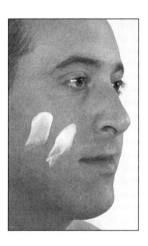

7. Wait five to fifteen minutes for the benzoyl peroxide to dry. You'll know the benzoyl peroxide is dry when your skin feels a bit tight and it may appear somewhat flaky. This is normal. Now apply the moisturizer. The moisturizer will take care of the tight-skin feeling and flakiness. You're the best judge of how much moisturizer to use. I

15 Minutes in the Morning

While you wait for your skin to dry after washing, or between your benzoyl peroxide and moisturizer applications, here are a few things you can do to utilize the time:

Read the newspaper. Make breakfast. Walk the dog. Blow-dry your hair. Check your email. Make your bed. Fold laundry. Empty the dishwasher. Write a letter.

The point is to create a ritual use of the time that helps you accomplish something while you wait, while keeping you on task as you apply the regimen.

apply slightly less moisturizer than benzoyl peroxide cream; use as much as you need to keep your skin from flaking during the day. If your skin is still flaky after a few minutes, apply more moisturizer. *Do not skip this step.* Begin moisturizing from day one. Apply the moisturizer as gently as you did the benzoyl peroxide.

Tips and Tricks

- Benzoyl peroxide can bleach fabrics, so don't wear your favorite shirt when applying it.
- Benzoyl peroxide can also bleach linens, so cover your pillows with old pillowcases to prevent damage to good ones.
- Wash your hands *very* well after applying benzoyl peroxide to prevent bleaching bathroom towels.
- Get even more out of an empty tube of benzoyl peroxide by cutting the tube in half and using your finger to scoop out what's left inside.
- Benzoyl peroxide can also bleach hair, so apply it carefully around the eyebrows and hairline.

Evening

The evening regimen closely follows the morning steps.

1. Gently splash your face, neck, and any other problem areas with warm water.

2. Generously lather up your hands with a gentle cleansing bar or wash.

3. To prep your skin for the benzoyl peroxide treatment, gently wash problem areas with your

hands, barely touching the skin. Don't rub or use a washcloth—it is too irritating. Rinse with warm water. Wash for only ten seconds to prevent skin irritation.

4. Gently pat dry with a towel.

5. Wait five to fifteen minutes for your skin to completely dry.

6. Wash and dry your hands.

7. Apply the benzoyl peroxide again to your problem areas, using the same guidelines for the amount of product to use outlined in the morning routine. Make sure to cover every inch, without rubbing too much. Do not skimp on the benzoyl peroxide once you get to week four and after!

8. As with the morning regimen, the amount of moisturizer to apply is up to you. If your skin feels dry and itchy from the regimen, even after you moisturize, use more, morning and night.

What Can I Expect as I Get Clear?

Everyone's skin will react differently when they begin using the Clear Skin regimen. However, I can give you some guidelines as to what you can expect for the first few weeks of the treatment, based on my personal experience and the feedback from others who have used the regimen to get clear.

IF YOU HAVE LIGHT ACNE

First week—Anywhere from slight improvement to dramatic clearing. Expect dryness and redness to the skin.

Second week—More clearing. May experience an unexpected breakout, but it should heal faster than it usually would. Expect continued dry and red skin.

Third week—Even more improvement. Skin starts to look smoother with many less pimples, if any. Dryness and redness begin to subside.

Fourth to Eighth weeks—Close to complete clearing if not totally clear. Dryness and redness should be gone.

Ninth week and beyond—Clear and staying clear, with continued maintenance of the regimen.

IF YOU HAVE MODERATE ACNE

First week—Slight improvement.

Second week—Further improvement followed by a breakout. The breakout clears faster than normal.

Third week—Continued clearing with occasional breakouts clearing quickly.

Fourth week—More improvement.

Fifth to Twelfth weeks—Acne continues to improve, perhaps with a few breakouts. These breakouts should heal quickly, so continue the regimen until (and after) total clearing is achieved.

Thirteenth week and beyond—Clear and staying clear, with continued maintenance of the regimen.

Those with light acne may experience clearing very quickly. Beginning with the smaller amount of benzoyl peroxide allows your skin to get used to it, so that by the time you've reached the full dosage, your skin is ready to be fully clear in the first one to two months.

Moderate acne can take up to a few months to clear, and relapses and breakouts may occur during the first two to three months. Don't worry, these breakouts will clear more quickly than they have in the past, and your skin will continue to become clearer as you maintain the regimen at the largest dosage.

Don't give up. Give the regimen at least one full month, preferably two, to judge its effectiveness. You may experience some breakouts during the clearing process, but don't lose heart. Once you've reached the point of using the full amount of benzoyl peroxide, don't let up on the application. I can't say this enough times: *Use plenty of benzoyl peroxide*—this is the key to the whole regimen. Be patient and use the regimen for two months, be strict and follow it precisely, and then judge how it works. Chances are you'll be amazed by what you see!

Razor Requirements ■

Make your razor regimen friendly. To prevent irritation, change the blade on your razor often—I change mine at least once a week. I am not a fan of electric razors because I have found them to be more irritating than blade shaving. The best razor I have ever tried is the Gillette Sensor Excel razor.

Shaving Tips for Men

It's not surprising that harsh razors and shave gels can wreak havoc on acne-prone skin. The key is to be gentle and choose the right products. Follow these steps for a non-irritating shave.

1. To get your beard razor ready, let the hot water in your shower splash on your face periodically while washing the rest of your body and shampooing your hair.

2. Vigorously lather up your hands with the cleansing bar and use the suds as shaving cream.

Spread on the thick lather using extremely gentle, circular motions. I recommend using only the lather from a cleansing bar to shave, but if you prefer to use a shaving gel or cream, read the label; purchase only those products that are non-comedogenic and oil-free, and which do not contain any acne-fighting ingredients.

3. Employ confident, downward strokes, going with the grain of your beard. You will likely want to shave the bottom part of your neck upward, as hair tends to reverse directions in that area. Avoid shaving over any area too many times. If you miss an area, though, just go back over it gently.

4. After you shave, lather up your hands again and wash your forehead, nose, and other problem areas gently.

5. Proceed with the morning steps of your Clear Skin regimen.

How often should you shave? Your best bet is to do it daily. The longer the facial hair growth between shaves, the more irritating the act of shaving itself is

Monthly Supply

As you've no doubt gathered by now, you're going to be using *a lot* of benzoyl peroxide, but how much is a lot? Here is an example of how much of each product you're going to be using on the Clear Skin regimen in one month:

- Benzoyl peroxide: four to eight 0.75-ounce tubes of On-the-Spot Acne Treatment
- Moisturizer: one 4-ounce container
- Cleanser: one bar for women, two bars for men (who shave with it)

Once you settle on a particular product that you're happy with, keep an eye out for sales so you can stock up. And check in with my website, www.acne.org, for updates as larger, more economical sizes become available.

to your skin. If you can shave every day, I highly recommend it.

Staying *Clear*

You made the commitment to get clear and now you are. Maintaining your Clear Skin means dedication to the Clear Skin regimen for the long haul. The maintenance regimen is exactly the same as it was for week four while you were getting clear. Follow the regimen precisely every day. *Continue to use a very generous amount of benzoyl peroxide. Every day. Without fail.* I can't emphasize this enough! Keeping your skin clear means not giving up on your fight against acne, and a lapse in your daily regimen can bring those pimples right back.

Daily Behaviors

The most important advice I can give you is to enjoy your day. I know what it's like to feel guilty for eating certain foods and worrying that stress from school or work is contributing to complexion problems. But no correlation has been found in studies attempting to link diet and acne. In other words, if you want that

Hershey bar, don't pass it up on that account! (If you are positive a certain food aggravates your acne, skip that food—but keep in mind that it is probably only a coincidence.) And don't stress about stress. Go about your daily activities assured that the benzoyl peroxide is working hard all day long.

Tweaking your daily habits can dramatically improve your acne. Even if you gave up harsh washcloths and vigorous scrubbing years ago, you may be unknowingly irritating your skin with other seemingly harmless habits. Try to avoid resting your chin in your hands, picking at your face, deeply burying your face in your pillow at night, and overwashing. Strive to leave your skin alone so it can get clear!

Cosmetics Conundrum

According to the National Institutes of Health, acne patients who use cosmetics should choose oil-free ones. I suggest avoiding cosmetics altogether if possible in the first weeks of the Clear Skin regimen. You want to give your skin the best possible chance to improve, and introducing any substance to your skin besides the three products used in the regimen (gentle cleanser, benzoyl peroxide, and moisturizer) may hinder your success.

If you must use cosmetics, understand that it may be difficult to apply foundation during the first few weeks of treatment because your skin may be red or scaly from the benzoyl peroxide. Use just a spot cover-up if you can, instead of an all-over foundation. Tinted On-the-Spot may be an option for that. If you feel you must use a cover-up or foundation on the whole face, at least take proper care when applying. Try to keep the process as clean as possible. When applying cosmetics with your fingers, make sure your hands are clean before you start. If applying with a cosmetic sponge or brush, be sure it is superclean. Oil can accumulate on sponges and brush bristles, so wash them once a week with your facial cleanser and let them air-dry overnight.

Beware, too, that hairstyling products that come in contact with the skin along your hairline can irritate your clearing skin, so apply them carefully.

When shopping for cosmetics that are touted as oil-free and non-comedogenic, be aware that the U.S. Food and Drug Administration does not regulate ingredients in cosmetics. Even though it's in the best interests of the cosmetics companies to provide products that truly are oil-free and non-comedogenic, it isn't always going to be so.

Now that you have the tools, you can begin your journey to Clear Skin! Take out your Skin Care Journal, write in today's date, and get started.

5

FREQUENTLY ASKED QUESTIONS

I am often asked questions about a whole lot of practical issues—from how skin reacts to benzoyl peroxide to acne maintenance to scar treatments. You're probably going to have lots of questions before you start, as well as during the course of the regimen, so here I'm answering the most frequently asked questions I've been asked at my website, providing answers from both my research and my own experience with acne and the Clear Skin regimen.

My skin is itchy after I apply the benzoyl peroxide. Is that normal?

A little itchiness is normal. This shouldn't last long,

just a couple of weeks while your skin is getting used to the benzoyl peroxide. Don't scratch in response to the itchiness. It will only irritate your skin and make your acne worse. Make sure you moisturize properly. It will help quite a bit.

My skin is burning and/or red after I apply the benzoyl peroxide. Is that normal?

A lot of people experience some redness when they begin the regimen. This usually subsides after a couple of weeks. If you have sensitive skin or start the regimen by using a lot of benzoyl peroxide, you should expect redness or dryness, sometimes severe. I strongly recommend starting with a lesser amount of benzoyl peroxide and increasing the amount over a period of a few weeks. If you experience severe burning, blistering, crusting, swelling, or skin rash, consult a physician right away.

My skin looks absolutely terrible. It is peeling off, red, and I am miserable. What do I do?

There are a couple of reasons for your severe skin reaction—you're either allergic to benzoyl peroxide or you started by using too much. About 3 percent of the population is allergic to benzoyl peroxide, so if you experience swelling, blistering, or crusting of the skin, stop using the product immediately. More likely the reason for your redness or dryness is that you just started by using too much product too quickly. It takes a while—from a few days to a few weeks—for your skin to get used to the benzoyl peroxide. If the condition really is too much for you, I suggest stopping the regimen completely to give your skin a week or two to recuperate. When you start up the regimen again, use a much smaller dosage of benzoyl peroxide to begin with, and increase the amount you use slowly to give your skin time to get used to it. You'll need to work up to the large amount of benzoyl peroxide in the regimen to attain total clearing.

My skin is dry from the benzoyl peroxide. Nothing can improve the dryness, even a lot of moisturizer. What do I do?
Alpha hydroxy moisturizers usually hydrate skin better than other moisturizers. But try an alpha hydroxy moisturizer only after a few weeks of being on the regimen, because it might sting if you use it at the beginning of the regimen.

Every once in a while I still get a pimple. What's up?

Realistically, you'll probably get a zit now and then—just like everybody does—while on the regimen. They should be rare and nothing to worry about. Just keep up with the regimen and don't give it a second thought.

The regimen is not working for me. What's going on?

Here are a few things to consider:

☐ Check the products you are using. Be sure you are using the oil-free, non-comedogenic products.

☐ Are you following the regimen *exactly?* Many people think they are, but they're not. For example, are you scrubbing your face too hard when washing? Are you still touching or picking at your face? Are you using enough benzoyl peroxide? Review the regimen again and compare it to what you're doing.

☐ Give the regimen one to two months to work. The acne you see in the first month might just be acne that was developing before you even started the regimen. Follow the treatment precisely for one to two months before you make a judgment.

☐ Have you been hanging out in the sun lately? Sun exposure can lead to breakouts, so the afternoon you spent in the sun three weeks ago could be the cause of your breakout today. Limit your sun exposure and use an SPF 15 moisturizer for further protection.

☐ As time goes on, people tend to start using less benzoyl peroxide and become less patient and precise in their application. Following the regimen in the beginning got you clear, so go back to the basics. Apply plenty of benzoyl peroxide gently and patiently.

The regimen worked, and I am clear now. Do I need to keep using the benzoyl peroxide?

Yes, keep going with the benzoyl peroxide and the regimen! Acne can't be cured, but it can be managed, so it's important to keep up with the regimen even after you get clear.

Is using benzoyl peroxide once a day enough?

No. This regimen works because you're applying the benzoyl peroxide twice a day. I've tried to do it only once daily, and it just doesn't produce the same results.

My skin isn't dry so I don't need to moisturize, right?

Wrong. You need to moisturize to keep your skin balanced. It is *very* important to moisturize whether you feel your skin is dry or not.

The moisturizer is balling up with the benzoyl peroxide. What's going on?

This may happen. Just gently brush the moisturizer–benzoyl peroxide residue off the surface of your skin with clean fingers. To prevent this in the future, try switching to a moisturizer that contains alpha hydroxy. This will work better with the benzoyl peroxide and should take care of the residue. Just make sure to wait to make the switch in moisturizers until you've been on the regimen for a few weeks. The alpha hydroxy may be too irritating to your skin when combined with the benzoyl peroxide in the beginning of the program.

Should I shave daily, every other day, or once a week?

The longer your facial hair grows, the more irritating shaving will be to the skin. Unless you have scant growth, I recommend shaving every day.

Can I use cosmetics? Which kinds are best?

If you can go cold turkey without cosmetics for the early weeks of the regimen, do it. If you can't, try to keep makeup to a minimum while you're getting clear in order to give the regimen time to work before introducing other products to your face. It may be hard to apply some foundations and/or cover-ups during the first few weeks of treatment because your skin can be dry and peeling. If you must wear makeup, look for cosmetics that are labeled *oil-free* and *non-comedogenic* and apply them gently.

Is it okay to get a tan in a tanning bed?

Not if you want to keep your acne under control.

Tanning beds damage skin and can irritate acne—just like the sun does—so don't use them.

Can I shower at night?

Sure. Just reverse the morning and evening routines.

I exercise during the day and sweat. Should I wash afterward? And what's up with the white residue on my face when I exercise?

Sweating and acne don't have anything to do with each other. The sweat glands are completely separate from the sebaceous glands (where acne develops); they open to the skin's surface in different places. Acne is formed well below the skin's surface, not from what's happening on top of the skin, so sweat just doesn't play a role. Since sweating doesn't affect the formation of acne, you don't have to wash again. Having said that, there is one exception. If you participate in sports where you wear a protective helmet or face mask that rubs against your skin or neck, you may want to consider washing your face following play and reapplying your benzoyl peroxide medication and moisturizer. The best thing to do, of course, is to schedule your exercise before your morning or evening routine to avoid the situation altogether. Whatever your exercise schedule, just be sure to do the regimen twice a day.

After exercising, you may see a white residue on the areas where you've applied the benzoyl peroxide. This is normal. Since it may take a while for all of the product to be fully absorbed into the skin, try to avoid exercising for a few hours after applying the benzoyl peroxide, or exercise in the morning or evening before you do the regimen. If you can't do this, blot the residue very lightly with a clean towel.

What do I do for bacne (acne on the back)?

The bottom line is that all light to moderate acne responds well to benzoyl peroxide treatments. Whether you've got acne on your face, back, neck, or chest, benzoyl peroxide is the way to go. Bacne can be treated with the Clear Skin regimen—gentle cleansing and lots of benzoyl peroxide. Apply the benzoyl peroxide in sections, just like you do to your face, because it's hard to cover such a large area all at once. You'll need a couple of good mirrors and flexible arms to apply benzoyl peroxide and moisturizer properly yourself! If there's someone you're comfortable asking for help, it might make the process easier.

Keep in mind that benzoyl peroxide can bleach fabric so treating your bacne can cost you a lot of clothes if you're not careful. If you're committed to clearing your bacne with the Clear Skin regimen, consider investing in a bunch of white T-shirts to wear alone or under other shirts to avoid bleaching out any colored clothes.

How do I get rid of the red marks after the blemish goes away?

According to the American Academy of Dermatology and Roche Laboratories, the red marks left after acne has healed aren't permanent. Time, of course, is the most effective treatment, as fading usually occurs within four to six months. These marks may appear as dark spots on darker-skinned people, but this isn't a scar either and will fade with time.

How do I get rid of scars?

There are different treatments for acne scars. The most common scar treatments are dermabrasion, laser resurfacing, chemical peels, punch techniques, subcision and augmentation. Each treatment is used for certain types of scars, so a thorough examination by a highly qualified and experienced dermatologist or cosmetic surgeon will help determine the procedure or combination of procedures that is right for you.

Can I use the Clear Skin regimen with the prescriptions I am currently taking?

Your doctor is really the person who should answer this question. Whether it's another acne medication you're taking or some other type of prescription, any side effects and possible drug interactions should be discussed with your doctor. Don't take any chances—check before you start the regimen.

Is benzoyl peroxide safe? Does it cause cancer?

Benzoyl peroxide is safe and has not been linked to cancer in humans. There was a study done in the early 1990s that showed benzoyl peroxide injected into mice with cancerous tumors increased the size of the tumors. After a short scare, this study was found to be uncontrolled and never could be duplicated. The

FDA unanimously voted to keep benzoyl peroxide available without a prescription.

Is it safe to use benzoyl peroxide while I'm pregnant?

No studies have been done on this subject. Check with your doctor before starting the Clear Skin regimen if you're pregnant or nursing.

I can't find the supplies in my area. Where can I order them?

For product delivery in the United States, you can order online at sites like www.drugstore.com. For people outside the United States, www.ShopInPrivate.com is one that offers international delivery. Products for the regimen are available at most independent drugstores and chain pharmacies.

Those small tubes of benzoyl peroxide are expensive. Where can I find a larger size?

Sometimes you can get a generic four-ounce tube of 2.5 percent benzoyl peroxide from a pharmacy with your health insurance coverage. Since this isn't an option for everyone, I recommend the smaller tube of

Neutrogena On-the-Spot Acne Treatment. I'm working with manufacturers to get them to make a larger,
more economical tube of benzoyl peroxide and I
won't rest until it's available to everyone. Check my
website (www.acne.org) for updates.

Do you know if the [Brand X] product is as good as the products you recommend?

No, I don't know if the Brand X product is as good as
the products I recommend. I do know from my experience in fighting acne all these years that the products
I recommend work. These products are gentle to
your skin and that's one of the main reasons they
work well within the Clear Skin regimen. However,
while I don't know personally if other brands work,
everyone's skin is different. If it's easier for you to
purchase a different product or you're curious about a
specific brand, it can't hurt to try it.

What about all of the other acne medications out there?

There are many products out there that treat acne—
from over-the-counter to prescription medications—
and I've tried just about all of them. Besides Accutane,

I haven't found anything that cleared up my acne better than benzoyl peroxide. Since Accutane comes with cautions of serious side effects, and even getting clear from it isn't a guarantee that you'll stay clear, benzoyl peroxide is the right medication to try first. It is widely available and, for people with light to moderate acne, it works. The Clear Skin regimen utilizes benzoyl peroxide to control your acne once and for all.

I hope that many of your questions have been answered in this chapter. It's important for you to understand that you're not alone in this fight against acne—lots of people have the same questions and are experiencing the same things that you are.

6

THE CLEAR PATH AHEAD

So, here we are. You've got the information, the product list, and the instructions, but you still may be a bit skeptical. After all, it sounds too easy and good to be true, right? Once again, I offer my own story as proof that this regimen can work for you. Just like you, I lived with acne for a long time and obsessed about every pimple. I tried all the "cures" out there and was elated when something would work for a while, but frustrated every time I broke out once again. That is, *until* I discovered this simple way to control my acne.

But don't rely on my word alone. There are people from all over the world who have tried the Clear

Skin method and finally found success in their battle with acne. Hundreds have written to tell me their own stories and how the Clear Skin method changed their lives. These are regular people—just like you and me—who came upon the Clear Skin method and thought, "Why not?"

Many of the people who offered the following testimonials showed remarkable improvement in their skin in just a short while. Some of these people probably started with the full blast of benzoyl peroxide, but this is *not* the best way for everyone. I strongly recommend starting off slowly with a small amount of benzoyl peroxide to give your skin time to get used to it and to reduce the occurrence of dry, red skin. Begin increasing the amount of benzoyl peroxide you use over a couple of weeks until you're using the full amount I've suggested. Don't worry—even beginning slowly you should still see dramatic results within about a month.

"As a person who has visited a dermatologist on a regular basis since the age of thirteen (I am now twenty-eight) it was difficult to believe this regimen would clear my skin in both an effective and an efficient manner. Three full weeks into the routine, my skin was 85 percent clear. At two months, my skin was 95 percent clear with a rare pimple or two. At three months, breakouts—major or minor—were nonexistent. I had no major problems with the regimen. My neck became slightly dry at first because this area had never been treated, but the moisturizer helped.

"In general, acne has been oftentimes quite painful and often distracting. I would develop some deep pimples on a nerve (under the skin) that would drive me crazy. Clearing my skin has given me peace of mind—from both pain and distraction."
—Anne

■　■　■

"My story is not unlike others. . . . I have battled acne for many years. It started to get bad when I turned fourteen. I am twenty now, and I spent my entire teenage years hating my face, trying to cover it with ugly thick makeup. I tried *everything*. My parents spent hundreds and hundreds of dollars on dermatologists, cleansers, 'miracle drugs,' . . . you name it, I've tried it. I have used Retin-A for six years now. I was just about ready to go on Accutane because this was the only choice I thought I had left . . . until I tried your simple solution. Within days, my face started clearing. It's been about a month and a

half now and my face continues to clear. It is amazing. I never thought I'd be able to go outside without makeup on. Thank you so much. You don't know how this has changed my life."
—Krystin

■ ■ ■

"Because it was so easy and cheap to try, I started the regimen immediately. Overnight, all my pimples scabbed up. In one week, my face was completely clear. It has been a little over a month and my face is still clear!" —Jacquelyn

■ ■ ■

"After trying for twenty years to clear up my skin I would have never thought such a simple and inexpensive regimen would work. I feel so much better about myself and how I look!!"
—Shelly

■ ■ ■

"I'm twenty-eight, and my skin has been giving me so many problems. I've been following your regimen and my face is clearing. People notice the difference! As you said, applying *a lot of benzoyl* is *the secret.* Thank you!!" —Sameera

■ ■ ■

"I've been using your method for five weeks and my acne has almost totally disappeared. Now I feel I can go out again without thinking people are just staring at my spots. I recommend this method to everyone with acne!" —Rich

■ ■ ■

"I have been following the regimen for two months now and my breakouts are over with. My skin is the clearest it has been since I was on Accutane but without the horrible dryness. I really can't praise your method enough." —Martin

■ ■ ■

"My daughter has had acne for about four years. She is eleven years old and she has been using [your method] for seventeen days now and I would say she is probably 75 percent cleared up. She says people do not call her zitface anymore." —Rose

■ ■ ■

"Your acne regimen works! I have suffered with acne for years. I started your regimen about two weeks ago and my face is so clear. I can't remember the last time my face was this clear. I no longer hide from mirrors." —Michael

■ ■ ■

"I started being plagued with acne fifteen years ago. I have tried dermatologists, and took antibiotics so long that I have become very resistant to many of them. At one point, my complexion was so bad just looking in the mirror without makeup made me cry. But just five weeks after starting your regimen, I went out for the *first* time in fifteen years today *without* makeup! I can't believe how *clear and soft* my skin is!"
—Angie

■ ■ ■

"I would like to thank you for the most incredible advice that I have ever received on clearing acne! It's hard to believe how simple this clearing routine [is] and the products used are so effective in clearing acne. I have been battling acne for twenty years and finally this routine has cleared my face!"
—Eddie

■ ■ ■

"My daughter started breaking out when she was eleven years old. The dermatologist started her on treatments of antibiotics and Retin-A with no improvement. The last treatment was a chemical peel that made her cry for days. I was excited to get my daughter started on [your] program. The results are no less than miraculous! It took about three weeks for the dramatic effects to take place. She ramped up slowly with the amount of [benzoyl peroxide] cream and she is almost completely clear now." —Maureen

■ ■ ■

"My wife and I tried a bunch of different things to help our son's acne problem but didn't have much luck. We followed your suggestions and in the last six months his face has cleared up and he has gained more self-esteem. Thank you very much." —John

■ ■ ■

"It's been a solid month and my skin is absolutely clear! It's soft and silky and makeup has once again become an accessory, not a camouflage." —Jessica

So what makes this regimen so special? Let's sum up what you've learned about acne and the Clear Skin method.

☐ Benzoyl peroxide will fight your acne. It is the most effective over-the-counter product for attacking the bacterium that promotes acne.

☐ Using a lower dosage of benzoyl peroxide provides the bacteria-killing benefits, but reduces the risk of overdrying, redness, and irritation you can experience with higher-dosage benzoyl peroxide products.

☐ Applying lots of benzoyl peroxide can get rid of existing pimples and keep you clear in the future.

☐ You must be gentle. This regimen emphasizes being gentle to your skin to help keep your acne at bay. The old myth that you can scrub away your acne just isn't true. In fact, it actually makes the situation worse. Be gentle during every phase of the regimen. Once you retrain yourself to think "gentle," your face will reward you with clearer skin.

☐ The Clear Skin regimen is simple and fits easily into your everyday life. The regimen can be done in just about fifteen to thirty minutes.

☐ You must stick to it. Once you get clear, you can't back off the fight. Remember, you can't *cure* acne, you can only *manage* it. You've got to continue with the regimen even after you get clear to stop future breakouts.

☐ You must protect yourself from sun exposure. The sun can aggravate your acne and cause flare-ups.

☐ Skin irritation can make acne worse. Don't touch or pick at your face. Be aware of helmet straps, tight collars, or even telephone handsets that rub against your skin and can cause irritation.

☐ It's not just what you put on your skin that will keep you clear. The total Clear Skin method is the combination of the Clear Skin regimen and modifying your behavior so you don't irritate your skin.

Here are some more people who have used the Clear Skin method and cleared up their skin. Look at the pictures, read their stories, and judge for yourself.

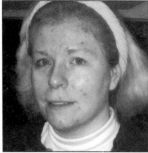
Chris Before

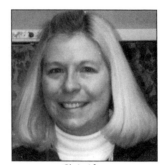
Chris After

"I never had acne until after my son was born. For three years I tried many products and shed many tears. Then I found Dan's regimen. It seemed easy. The products are readily available and fairly inexpensive, considering everything I had already tried. My skin is very fair and equally sensitive. I went through the hardening effect for three to four weeks. I could not wear makeup during this time. It would just clump up on my face. Also, in my experience, my face was never red and I cleared up in about two weeks. Like anyone, I still get an occasional pimple. However, I am *so* thankful for Dan! I have my confidence back!" —Chris

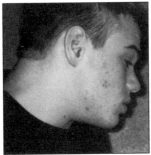

Patrick Before

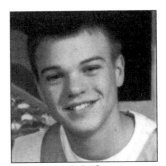

Patrick After

"When I began the acne regimen, I really did not expect much—just fewer bad blemishes. After about one week, my skin became very dry and uncomfortable. At the same time, I was not getting any more new 'bad' areas. As long as I used a lot of the moisture cream, I didn't flake, so it was okay. In about three weeks I really noticed my skin clearing up all over. It felt great to be thirteen!" —Patrick

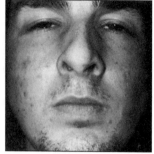
Keith Before

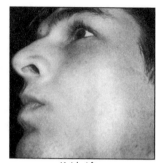
Keith After

"This regimen is nothing less than amazing. I've battled with acne ever since I was a young teenager, and I was losing. I hated my face. Having tried so many other medications, I was skeptical when I learned of this regimen. It's so simple, and you can't beat the cost, so I gave it a try. I couldn't believe how well it worked. I had a little bit of dryness at first, but my face was getting clear—and fast. Three weeks later my face was nearly clear. My confidence has gone way up because of this regimen. I only wish I had learned of it sooner!!" —Keith

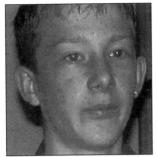
Tim N. Before

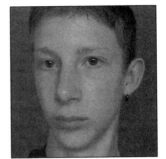
Tim N. After

"My experience with the regimen has led me to believe that miracles are indeed possible. The incapability of clearing up acne is extremely frustrating and demeaning. After finally finding and beginning the regimen, my skin went from bad to worse for about two days. At the beginning my skin was very red and dry, but after a few days I was fairly comfortable and those symptoms were no longer a problem. After that, it was uphill. It didn't take long for noticeable results, and new acne became a rarity. After about two to four months I was almost completely clear, and it was maybe another month before it was all entirely gone. With my confidence through the roof, it was much easier to engage in social activity. The burden of embarrassment and self-consciousness was alleviated, and things have only gotten better. The regimen has changed my life in more ways than one, and for that, I am thankful." —Tim N.

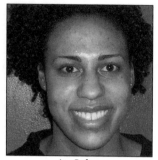
Joy Before

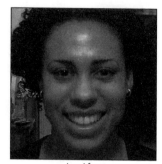
Joy After

"I have had persistent, moderate acne since I was thirteen. I tried everything for twelve years—over-the-counter medications, dermatologist prescriptions like Retin-A and antibiotics, even ProActiv and restrictive diets. *Nothing worked!* I constantly felt embarrassed and self-conscious about my skin. It was hard to socialize. I thought about my acne constantly. I avoided cameras. In three weeks of using Dan's regimen I saw a big difference. In six weeks I was totally clear! It has completely changed the way I see myself. I feel more confident, secure, and beautiful. I will always be grateful to Dan for changing my life!" —Joy

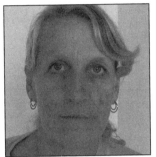
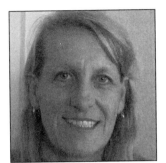

Claudia Before   Claudia After

"My face started to clear within three days of starting the regimen. Active acne spots started to dry up, and gently sloughed off. I have always had an underlying red blotchiness to my skin, and that faded dramatically within the first month. I think the keys to the regimen for me were to wash and touch my face as gently as possible, and to apply all three elements to my nose last.

"I do a considerable amount of public speaking, and my acne was a real stress point for me. I have been in business for twenty-five years and feel more self-confident in public now than I ever did. The regimen has been a huge boon to me."
—Claudia

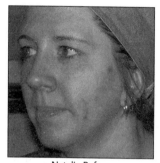
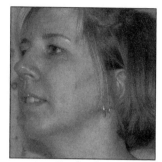

Natalie Before   Natalie After

"I've never used a 2.5 percent benzoyl peroxide before this regimen. I've only used a 10 percent with much dryness and little benefit. I was amazed what I saw in just the use of 2.5 percent benzoyl peroxide. I used a large amount as told. I never would have thought to do this on my own. Every day I'm clearer and my scars are lessened daily too. I've had *no* dryness—in fact, less than ever before. Now I actually go out without makeup on, which may not seem like a big deal, but I'm thirty and have worn makeup since I was twelve. Now I just don't have anything to cover up!" —Natalie

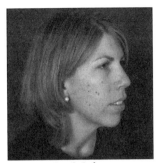

Ann S. Before

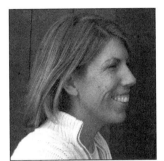

Ann S. After

"Once I started the regimen, it took about a week or so to really see the results. I found the regimen effective and easy to follow. The only problem I experienced was a bit of dryness in the beginning. However, it went away after a short period of time and has been fine ever since.

"Before I started this regimen it was very obvious that I had an acne problem. Within a week, people started telling me how great I looked and asking me what I was doing to make my skin look so fresh and vibrant. A few people even asked if I had gotten a new hairstyle or changed something about my look because they said I looked so good!" —Ann S.

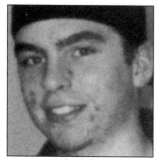

Dylan Before

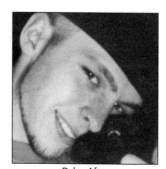

Dylan After

"I had acne for several years. It was a horrible experience that I would not wish on anyone. When I started the regimen, I did not expect it to work. After all, why should it? Nothing else had. I was very happily surprised to see my face clear up dramatically in a matter of weeks. The only side effect I incurred was slightly dry skin. This is a side effect of most acne treatments, so it was nothing I was not prepared for. I finally found the solution to my problem!" —Dylan

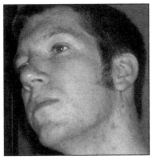

Tim S. Before

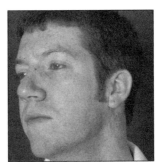

Tim S. After

"The regimen worked so wonderfully for me. I noticed my skin improving after the first week. After suffering from acne for most of my life, I was nothing short of amazed at the effectiveness of this treatment. The incorporation of an oil-free moisturizer into the process completely offset the only potential 'side effect,' which would be dry skin. After months of following the regimen, I no longer have acne and my confidence level has never been higher. As a lifelong skeptic, I will back this process wholeheartedly. Why? Because it works!" —Tim S.

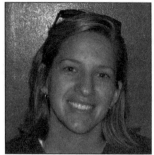
Ann M. Before

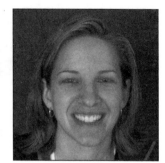
Ann M. After

"I am a twenty-two-year-old collegiate athlete and have had acne for about six years. After trying tetracycline, Differin gel, BenzaClin, ProActiv, and many other over-the-counter solutions, I became very frustrated. I went searching for a solution to moderate acne and found Dan's regimen. After only one week of using the Purpose cleansing bar, Neutrogena On-the-Spot treatment, and Neutrogena moisturizer, I could tell my skin was more smooth and I had fewer breakouts. It took about four weeks until I had consistently clear skin. I am committed to this regimen because it works!" —Ann M.

These are the pictures and stories of just some of the people who have used the Clear Skin regimen and found success in their battle with acne. They give you the true lowdown on their experiences as examples of what you may encounter using the regimen, or your way to becoming clear.

The regimen is different from any other method out there because it gives you all of the information to help you get clear and stay clear. You don't just get a bunch of products and let loose on your skin—you know *exactly* how and why to do everything it takes to get clear. This step-by-step regimen leaves no doubt—follow the directions exactly and it will clear your acne. Through all the years of trying just about every acne treatment available, no one ever nailed down precisely *how* to clear up my skin. It isn't just about the products—it's how you treat your skin as well. This is what makes the Clear Skin regimen different and what will make it work for you.

Skin Care Journal

WEEK #:

DAY:

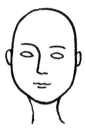

To get an accurate sense of what percentage of your face acne is affecting, study your skin carefully in a mirror. Sketch onto the drawing where you have blemishes on your face and neck.

How did your skin react to the benzoyl peroxide today? Did it become dry or itchy? How does it feel to the touch?

What improvements did you notice today?

INDEX

Page numbers in *italic* indicate illustrations.

Accutane treatment, 5–6, 6–7, 79–80

Acne, xi–9

    Accutane treatment, 5–6, 6–7, 79–80

    antibiotic treatment, 4

    benzoyl peroxide, xii–xiii, 4, 5, 7–8, 9, 39–40

    clindamycin treatment, 6

    Daniel Kern's story, xi, xii, 3–9, 46

    disease, acne as a, xi–xii, 23

    dry skin from treatments, 5, 6, 7, 8

    gentle treatment of skin and, 4–5, 41, 89–90

    grades of, xii

    lesion number and grade of, xii

    moisturizers, 6, 7, 8

    over-the-counter treatment, xii–xiii

    Retin-A treatment, 4

    scarring from, 27, 29, 76–77

    severe (cystic) acne, xii, 19, 25, 26–27

    sulfur treatment, 6

    washing face and, 4–5, 8, 29, 33

    See also Biology behind acne; Clear Skin; Emotions surrounding acne; Factors that worsen acne; Myths of acne

Acne conglobata, xii

Acne cosmetica, xii

Acne mechanica, xi–xii

Acne tropicalis, xii

Acne vulgaris (common acne), xii

Adolescence and acne, 28

Adulthood and acne, 28

Allergies to benzoyl peroxide, 44, 69

Alpha hydroxy moisturizers, 45, 72–73

American Academy of Dermatology, 76

Amounts of products, monthly, 60
Anger from acne, 14
Antibiotic treatment, 4
Antidepressants, acne worsening from, 31

Babies and acne, 28
Back acne (bacne), 75–76
Bacteria *(Propionibacterium acnes),* 24, 41
Basis products, 45
Benzoyl peroxide
 allergies to, 44, 69
 cancer from, 77–78
 Clear Skin regimen and, 41–42, 44, 57, 89
 dosage of, 44, 89
 expense of, 46, 60, 78–79
 health insurance for, 78
 history of acne treatment, xii–xiii, 4, 5, 7–8, 9, 39–40
 insurance coverage for, 78
 monthly supply, 60
 over-the-counter, 46
 oxygen, benefits of, 41
 percentages of, 41–42, 44, 46
 pregnancy, 78
 safety of, 77–78
 tips and tricks, 53
Biology behind acne, 23–35
 adolescence and acne, 28
 adulthood and acne, 28
 babies and acne, 28
 bacteria *(Propionibacterium acnes),* 24, 41
 blackheads (comedones), xii, 19, 25, 26
 blocked pores and acne, 24, 25
 boils vs. acne, 27
 cysts, xii, 19, 25, 26–27
 dominant gene of acne, 28

hair follicles (pores) and acne, 24, 25
 heredity as indicator for, 28
 nodules, xii, 19, 25, 26–27
 pores (blocked) and acne, 24, 25
 rashes vs. acne, 27
 red bumps (papules), xii, 19, 25, 26
 red rimmed whiteheads (pustules), xii, 19, 25, 26
 rosacea vs. acne, 27
 sebaceous glands, 24
 sebum (oil), 24, 25
 start of acne, 24, 25
 whiteheads (comedones), xii, 19, 25
 See also Acne; Clear Skin; Factors that worsen acne; Myths of acne
Blackheads (comedones), xii, 19, 25, 26
Blocked pores and acne, 24, 25
Boils vs. acne, 27
Brands recommended, 45–46, 79
Burning, 68

Cancer from benzoyl peroxide, 77–78
Cetaphil products, 45
Chopra, Deepak, 20
Cleansers, 43–44, 60
Clear path ahead, 83–103, *92–102*
Clear Skin Frequently Asked Questions, 67–80
 allergies to benzoyl peroxide, 44, 69
 alpha hydroxy moisturizers, 45, 72–73
 back acne (bacne), 75–76
 burning, 68
 cancer from benzoyl peroxide, 77–78
 cosmetics, 73
 dryness, 69
 exercising, 74–75

expense of benzoyl peroxide, 46, 60, 78–79

health insurance and benzoyl peroxide, 78

itchiness, 67–68

Maintenance Regimen, 71–72

medications for acne vs. Clear Skin, 79–80

medications with Clear Skin regimen, 77

moisturizers, 72–73

no results from regimen, 70–71

occasional pimple, 70

once daily vs. twice daily, 72

pregnancy and benzoyl peroxide, 78

prescriptions and Clear Skin, 77

product availability, 78

red marks left after acne, 76

redness, 68

safety of benzoyl peroxide, 77–78

scar treatments, 76–77

severe skin reaction, 68–69

shaving, 57–59, 73

showering at night, 74

tanning, 73–74

Clear Skin regimen, 39–63, 83–103

alpha hydroxy moisturizers, 45, 72–73

amounts of products, monthly, 60

brands recommended, 45–46, 79

cleansers, 43–44, 60

cosmetics (oil-free and non-comedogenic), 62–63, 73

daily behaviors, 61

dosage of benzoyl peroxide, 44, 89

Evening Regimen, 52–54, 74

formula, 40–41

gentle cleansing, 4–5, 41, 89–90

hairstyling products, 63

journaling progress, 46, 104–9, *104–9*

light acne, 19, 25, 55, 56

Maintenance Regimen, 59–60, 71–72

mild acne, 19, 25, 55, 56

moderate acne, 19, 25, 55–56, 56–57

moisturizers, 8, 41, 43, 45, 60, 72–73

monthly supply of products, 60

Morning Regimen, 47–52, *48–49, 51,* 74

oxygen of benzoyl peroxide, benefits of, 41

percentages of benzoyl peroxide, 41–42, 44, 46

product checklist, 43–46

razors for shaving, 58

recommended brands, 45–46, 79

results, expectations, 54–57

ritual use of time, 52

shaving tips for men, 57–59, 73

Skin Care Journal, 46, 104–9, *104–9*

SPF with moisturizer, 43, 45

starting, 44, 46

summary of, 89–91

testimonials, 84–89, *92–102, 92–103*

time for, 54–57

tips and tricks, 53

Website for, 46, 60, 78

See also Acne; Benzoyl peroxide; Clear Skin Frequently Asked Questions

Clindamycin treatment, 6

Comedogenic cosmetics, xii, 32

Comedones (blackheads, whiteheads), xii, 19, 25, 26

Common acne *(acne vulgaris),* xii

INDEX

Cosmetics
  comedogenic, xii, 32
  oil-free and non-comedogenic,
    62–63, 73
Cystic (severe) acne, xii, 19, 25,
  26–27

Daily behaviors, 61
Depression from acne, 14–15
Desperation from acne, 15–16
Diet as cause of acne (myth), 32–33,
  61
Disease, acne as a, xi–xii, 23. *See also*
  Biology behind acne
Dominant gene of acne, 28
Dosage of benzoyl peroxide, 44, 89
Drugstore.com, 78
Dryness from Clear Skin, 69
Dry skin from acne treatments, 5, 6, 7,
  8

Emotions surrounding acne, 13–19
  anger, 14
  depression, 14–15
  desperation, 15–16
  frustration, 16–17
  "I'll try anything" response, 15–16
  negative self-image, 17
  overview of, 3, 13
  resignation, 17–18
  self-consciousness, 18
  self-image, negative, 17
  See also Acne; Clear Skin
Environmental irritants, acne
  worsening from, xii, 31
Eucerin products, 45
Evening Regimen, 52–54, 74
Exercising, 74–75
Expense of benzoyl peroxide, 46, 60,
  78–79

Factors that worsen acne, 28–32
  antidepressants, 31
  cosmetics (comedogenic), xii, 32
  environmental irritants, xii, 31
  friction, xi–xii, 30–31
  hands on face, 31
  harsh washclothes, 4–5, 29
  hormonal changes, 30
  hormone medications, 31
  hot, humid climates and acne, xii,
    31
  irritating skin, 4–5, 9, 29, 33
  lithium, 31
  mechanical friction, xi–xii, 30–31
  medications, 31
  picking, 29–30
  washing harshly, 4–5, 29, 33
  See also Biology behind acne
FAQs (Frequently Asked Questions).
  See Clear Skin Frequently Asked
  Questions
FDA (U.S. Food and Drug
  Administration), 63, 78
Formula of Clear Skin, 40–41
Frequently Asked Questions (FAQs).
  See Clear Skin Frequently Asked
  Questions
Friction, acne worsening from, xi–xii,
  30–31
Frustration from acne, 16–17

Gentle cleansing, 4–5, 41, 89–90
Gillette Sensor Excel, 58
Grades of acne, xii

Hair follicles (pores) and acne, 24, 25
Hairstyling products, 63
Hands on face, acne worsening from,
  31
Harsh washclothes, 4–5, 29

Health insurance and benzoyl peroxide, 78

Heredity as indicator for acne, 28

Hormonal changes, acne worsening from, 30

Hormone medications, acne worsening from, 31

Hot, humid climates, acne worsening from, xii, 31

"I'll try anything" response, 15–16

Insurance coverage for benzoyl peroxide, 78

Irritating skin, acne worsening from, 4–5, 9, 29, 33

Itchiness, 67–68

Journaling progress, 46, 104–9, *104–9*

Kern, Daniel, xi, xii, 3–9, 46

Lesion number and grade of acne, xii

Light acne, 19, 25, 55, 56. *See also* Clear Skin

Lithium, acne worsening from, 31

Maintenance Regimen, 59–60, 71–72

Masturbation as cause of acne (myth), 34

Mechanical friction, acne worsening from, xi–xii, 30–31

Medications
  acne worsening from, 31
  Clear Skin, using with, 77
  Clear Skin vs., 79–80

Mild acne, 19, 25, 55, 56. *See also* Clear Skin

Moderate acne, 19, 25, 55–56, 56–57. *See also* Clear Skin

Moisturizers
  Clear Skin Frequently Asked Questions, 72–73
  Clear Skin regimen and, 41, 43, 45
  history of acne treatment, 6, 7, 8
  monthly supply, 60

Monthly supply of products, 60

Morning Regimen, 47–52, *48–49, 51,* 74

Myths of acne, 32–35
  diet as cause of acne, 32–33, 61
  masturbation as cause of acne, 34
  sex as cause of acne, 34
  stress as cause of acne, 33–34, 61
  sun exposure can help acne, 34–35
  washing face more will cure acne, 33
  See also Biology behind acne

National Institutes of Health, 62

Negative self-image, 17

Neutrogena products, 45, 46, 62, 79

Nodules, xii, 19, 25, 26–27

Non-comedogenic cosmetics, 62–63, 73

No results from regimen, 70–71

Occasional pimple, 70

Oil-free and non-comedogenic cosmetics, 62–63, 73

Oil (sebum), 24, 25

Once daily vs. twice daily, 72

On-the-Spot Acne Treatment (Neutrogena), 46, 62, 79

Over-the-counter treatment, xii–xiii, 46

Oxy 10, 10

Oxygen of benzoyl peroxide, benefits of, 41

Papules (red bumps), xii, 19, 25, 26
Percentages of benzoyl peroxide,
    41–42, 44, 46
Picking pimples, 29–30
Pimples. *See* Acne
Pores (blocked) and acne, 24, 25
Pregnancy and benzoyl peroxide, 78
Prescriptions and Clear Skin, 77
Product availability, 78
Product checklist, 43–46
Propionibacterium acnes, 24, 41
Purpose products, 45
Pustules (red rimmed whiteheads), xii,
    19, 25, 26

Questions. *See* Clear Skin Frequently
    Asked Questions

Rashes vs. acne, 27
Razors for shaving, 58
Recommended brands, 45–46, 79
Red bumps (papules), xii, 19, 25, 26
Red marks left after acne, 76
Redness, 68
Red rimmed whiteheads (pustules),
    xii, 19, 25, 26
Resignation from acne, 17–18
Results, expectations, 54–57
Retin-A treatment, 4
Ritual use of time, 52
Roche Laboratories, 76
Rosacea vs. acne, 27

Safety of benzoyl peroxide, 77–78
Scarring from acne, 27, 29
Scar treatments, 76–77

Sebaceous glands, 24
Sebum (oil), 24, 25
Self-consciousness from acne, 18
Self-image, negative, 17
Severe (cystic) acne, xii, 19, 25, 26–27
Severe skin reaction, 68–69
Sex as cause of acne (myth), 34
Shaving, 57–59, 73
ShopInPrivate.com, 78
Showering at night, 74
Skin Care Journal, 46, 104–9, *104–9*
SPF with moisturizer, 43, 45
Starting Clear Skin, 44, 46
Start of acne, 24, 25
Stress as cause of acne (myth), 33–34,
    61
Sulfur treatment, 6
Summary of Clear Skin regimen,
    89–91
Sun exposure can help acne (myth),
    34–35

Tanning, 73–74
Testimonials, 84–89, *92–102,* 92–103
Time, ritual use of, 52
Time for Clear Skin, 54–57
Tips and tricks, 53

U.S. Food and Drug Administration
    (FDA), 63, 78

Washing face and acne, 4–5, 8, 29, 33
Website for Clear Skin, 46, 60, 78
Whiteheads (comedones), xii, 19, 25

Zits. *See* Acne